Bipolar Disorder

Bipolar Disorder Types, Diagnosis, Symptoms, Treatment,
Causes,
Effects, Prognosis, Research,
History, Myths, and More!

By Frederick Earlstein

Foreword

Bipolar Disorder, believe it or not, has been around since the ancient times! This disorder is one of the most common types of neurological condition that still exists today.

According to the National Institute of Mental Health (NIMH), bipolar disorder in United States alone affects around 2% of adults, and nearly 80% of them have been diagnosed as a severe case. Unfortunately lots of people (about 60%) are not receiving proper treatment due to many issues such as lack of awareness and knowledge about the disorder, financial incapacity, or social stigma.

Fortunately, bipolar disorder is highly treatable. If you or any of your friends and family is suffering from such illness, it is better gain some knowledge about this condition, so that you'll know how to combat it, and also be able to help others who are suffering from it. This book will provide you with a wealth of information about bipolar disorder; what it is, its effects, its treatment, and how to deal with it.

Table of Contents

Introduction

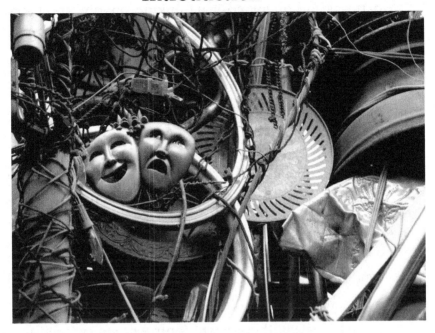

Bipolar disorder was also known as manic depression. It is a kind of mental health disorder that causes a person to have emotional mood swings that are usually extreme – either a person becomes depress (emotional low) or becomes emotionally manic (hypomania/high). A person with a bipolar disorder can either suffer from depression for a certain period of time and then suddenly shifts to a feeling of euphoria or too much happiness, then shifts again to feeling sad – and vice – versa. Their ever changing environment highly affects their emotional state.

Bipolar disorder also affects a person's sleeping patterns, judgment, critical thinking, energy, and behavior. They can suddenly lose interest for no reason, or become hopeless over something, sometimes it's the opposite they can be so happy and full of energy for no reason too! That's precisely why it's called bipolar – they shift from one extreme mood to another.

Mood swings usually occur multiple times in a year, for some people it just happens occasionally. Emotional symptoms may not be experienced by some people in between episodes. Even though bipolar disorder is a condition that a person needs to endure for his/her lifetime, it is manageable, and treatable. Proper medications can be given by psychotherapist to control mood swings, and this neurological condition can be improved through counseling.

This book contains some of the basic information regarding bipolar disorder: its history, the myths surrounding it, its different types, the different symptoms, treatments, diagnosis, and prognosis. We also look at some of the alternative or complementary treatments available, as well as some unconventional recommendations you can try.

Glossary

Acute: Relatively short but severe, as in an acute mood episode.

Adjunctive: Complementary to the main treatment.

Affective disorder: A category of psychiatric disorders that includes depression, bipolar disorder, and seasonal affective disorder (SAD). Affect is a medical term for mood.

Akathisia: Severe restlessness, a possible side effect of certain medications, especially some antipsychotics.

Anticonvulsant: A class of medications developed primarily to prevent epileptic seizures. Many anticonvulsants, including valproate (Depakote) and carbamazepine (Tegretol), are also useful in treating mania.

Antidepressant: A class of medications effective in treating the symptoms of depression.

Antipsychotic: A class of medications originally developed to reduce the frequency and severity of psychotic episodes. The newer atypical or second-generation antipsychotics are now also used to treat bipolar disorder or more severe depression. Many people who take these medications don't have psychotic symptoms.

Bipolar disorder: A psychiatric condition characterized by extreme mood states of mania and depression. A person may have bipolar disorder even if he has experienced only one of the extreme mood states, making diagnosis very challenging.

Bipolar I: A type of bipolar disorder characterized by at least one full-blown manic episode that doctors can't attribute to another cause, such as a medication or substance abuse. A bipolar I diagnosis doesn't require an episode of major depression, although periods of mania often alternate with periods of depression.

Bipolar II: A type of bipolar disorder characterized by at least one major depressive episode that doctors can't attribute to another cause, along with one or more hypomanic episodes. The depression tends to be chronic and is usually more problematic than the hypomania.

Some people with bipolar II develop a full manic episode, which changes the diagnosis to bipolar I.

Bipolar NOS (not otherwise specified): A type of bipolar disorder listed in the fourth edition of Diagnostic and Statistical Manual of Mental Disorders (DSM-IV) that's characterized by hypomanic, manic, or depressive episodes that don't fit in any of the other bipolar categories and can't be ascribed to unipolar depression.

Catatonia: A state of profound lack of movement and language, often including odd or unusual physical and verbal responses to stimuli. Sometimes alternates with periods of agitation and overexcitement, can be associated with bipolar disorder, unipolar depression, schizophrenia, and other psychiatric and medical conditions.

Circadian rhythm: An individual's biological pattern of sleep, wakefulness, and energy that plays out through the course of a day. Some studies show that irregularities in a person's circadian rhythm can destabilize moods.

Cognitive behavioral therapy (CBT): A therapy that works at the intersection between thoughts, feelings, and behavior. It is an active process; the therapist teaches about concepts and strategies, and the patient practices new skills outside of the sessions. Many studies show that CBT is effective for treating depression, anxiety, obsessive compulsive disorder, insomnia, PTSD, and some pain syndromes. Researchers are studying its use in other conditions as well.

Comorbid: Any medical condition that presents along with and often independent from another condition. People who have bipolar disorder can have other comorbid conditions — such as attention deficit hyperactivity disorder (ADHD), alcoholism, or anxiety disorder — that complicate the diagnosis and treatment of bipolar disorder.

Cyclothymia: Sometimes referred to as bipolar lite, a muted form of bipolar that nevertheless interferes with a person's life. It involves multiple episodes of hypomania and depressive symptoms that don't meet the criteria for mania or major depression. Symptoms must last for at least two years, (one year in children and teens) during which time there are no more than two symptom-free months.

De-compensation: The return of symptoms that had been under control, relapse.

Deep brain stimulation (DBS): Electronic stimulation of targeted areas of the brain that has been shown in some studies to reduce the symptoms of treatment resistant depression (TRD).

Diagnostic and Statistical Manual of Mental Disorders (DSM): A book that describes the criteria for diagnosing various mental illnesses and related conditions and that psychiatrists in the United States refer to when developing a diagnosis. DSM is similar to the International Classification of Diseases (ICD) used in most countries outside the United States.

Differential diagnosis: The process of distinguishing between two or more diseases or conditions that feature identical or similar symptoms. A doctor commonly performs a differential diagnosis to rule out other possibilities.

Dopamine: Often described as a feel-good neurotransmitter, dopamine is linked to feelings of pleasure and reward. It modulates attention, focus, and muscle movements, is involved in addiction, and is related to psychosis.

Dysthymia: Chronic, low-level depression that's commonly characterized by irritability and an inability to feel pleasure or joy. In DSM-5, now described as persistent depressive disorder.

Electroconvulsive therapy (ECT): A medical procedure in which a low-level electrical current is applied to the brain to induce a mild seizure in order to treat severe depression. ECT is often successful in treating depression that doesn't respond to medicine or therapy or when patients have had intolerable side effects with medicines or have medical conditions that prevent them from taking antidepressants.

ECT can also be an effective treatment for mania and catatonia.

Epigenetics: The study of the changes that affect the expression of genes but don't change the genes themselves.

Essential fatty acid (EFA): A healthy fat that the body uses for tissue development and other purposes and that must be obtained through diet. Omega-3 is a source of several EFAs that may be valuable in treating many health problems, including mood disorders.

Euthymic: Moods considered being in the normal range — not manic or depressive.

Executive function: The ability to organize, sort, and manage internal and external stimuli and generate adaptive and effective responses. Many psychiatric disorders weaken executive functioning, often leading to impaired judgment and uninhibited speech or behavior.

Expressed emotion: A term used by researchers to describe expressions of criticism or conflict that can have negative effects on people with mood disorders or other mental illness.

Gamma-aminobutyric acid (GABA): An amino acid neurotransmitter that works mostly as an inhibitor or calming-down agent in the brain.

Glutamate: A neurotransmitter that's involved in revving up the central nervous system. Glutamate circuits may play a significant role in the development of mania and depression.

G-protein-linked receptors: These are also called metabotropic receptors, and are one of two main types of receptors found on cell surfaces, G-protein-linked receptors are part of a signal system that communicates between chemicals outside of the cell, including neurotransmitters such as serotonin. These chemicals attach to the G-protein-linked receptors, triggering specific reactions inside the cell. These systems have been linked to the development of mood symptoms and to many of the medications used to treat bipolar disorder.

Hypersexual: Having an excessive interest or involvement in sexual activity.

Hyperthymic: A medical term for high energy sometimes used to describe a personality profile that includes being highly extroverted, very active physically and mentally, highly confident, temperamental, stimulus seeking, and risk taking.

Hypomania: An elevated mood that doesn't qualify as full-blown mania but typically involves increased energy, less need for sleep, clarity of vision, and a strong creative drive. These changes are noticeable to others but don't significantly impair daily function.

Insight: A clear acceptance and understanding of a psychological disorder and the ability to objectively observe one's own behaviors and attitudes that are characteristic of the disorder.

International Classification of Diseases (ICD): The diagnostic manual developed by the World Health

Organization (WHO) and used in most countries outside the United States. The ICD includes a chapter on the Classification of Mental and Behavioral Disorders, which is similar to the Diagnostic and Statistical Manual of Mental Disorders (DSM) used in the United States.

Interpersonal and social rhythm therapy (IPSRT): A therapy developed to maintain mood stability through strict scheduling, learning about personal roles, coping with transitions, developing healthy routines, increasing social contact, and resolving and preventing interpersonal problems.

Maintenance dose: An amount of a prescription medication that's intended to prevent the onset of symptoms rather than treat existing symptoms.

Major depressive episode: An extreme low mood that lasts at least two weeks and is characterized by symptoms such as despair, fatigue, loss or increase in appetite, loss of interest in pleasurable activities, an increased need for sleep or inability to sleep, and thoughts of death or suicide.

Mania: An extremely elevated mood typically characterized by euphoria, excessive energy, impulsivity, nervousness, impaired judgment, irritability, and a decreased need for sleep.

Manic depression: Another name for bipolar disorder.

Manic episode: A period of elevated mood, euphoric or irritable, typically characterized by impulsivity, nervousness, impaired judgment, irritability, and a decreased need for sleep. The period must last at least one week (or shorter if it leads to hospitalization).

MAOI (monoamine oxidase inhibitor): A class of antidepressant medications that slow the action of monoamine oxidase, an enzyme responsible for breaking down dopamine, serotonin, and norepinephrine in the brain. Because of the strict diet changes needed when taking MAOIs, doctors typically prescribe them only if a person reacts poorly to other antidepressants.

Mechanism of action: The way a medication acts on the biology or physiology of the brain to produce the desired effect.

Mindfulness: A mental state of focusing on the present moment, creating active awareness of internal and external experiences, with full acceptance and without judgment. Mindfulness can be practiced in many ways, including particular types of meditation. Numerous scientific studies support the cognitive, emotional, and behavioral benefits of a variety of mindfulness strategies.

Mood chart: A graph that shows the rise and fall of mood levels over time. Mood charts are very useful in predicting the onset of mood episodes and documenting the response to medications.

Mood disorder: A psychiatric condition that results in persistently disrupted moods and/or mood regulation.

Mood stabilizer: Strictly speaking, a medication that reduces frequency and/or severity of episodes of depression and/ or mania. The term has become commonly, if inaccurately, associated with any medications that have anti-manic effects or that reduce agitation.

Neuroleptic: Another name for antipsychotics, neuroleptics led the charge in pharmacological treatment of mental illness in the 1950s and 1960s.

Neuroleptic malignant syndrome: A potentially fatal but very rare side effect of antipsychotic medications that results in high temperature, muscle rigidity, and altered consciousness.

Neurons: Cells that are part of the telecommunications network in the brain and other parts of the nervous system; they carry signals throughout the body.

Neuroplasticity: The ability of the nervous system to adapt in response to internal and external stimuli or events. Some treatments for bipolar disorder appear to affect the capacity for change and growth in the nervous system.

Neurotransmitter: A chemical that's part of the communication systems between cells within the nervous system and from the nervous system to other parts of the body.

Norepinephrine: Best known for its role in the fight-or-flight response, norepinephrine is a neurotransmitter that functions to regulate mood, anxiety, and memory.

Off-label: A legal and legitimate use of a prescription medication to treat symptoms that the FDA (Food and Drug Administration) in the United States or comparable agencies in other countries didn't officially approve it to treat.

Omega-3: A source of several essential fatty acids that some experts believe is vital to the healthy development and function of the brain. Omega-3 is present in high concentration in cold-water ocean fish, including sardines, herring, and salmon; walnuts; flaxseed; and supplements.

Other specified bipolar and related disorders: One of the DSM-5 categories of bipolar disorder, replacing bipolar disorder NOS in the DSM–IV. This category relates to someone with most, but not all, of the symptoms of a specific type of bipolar; for example, all of the symptoms of hypomania but not lasting the necessary duration of four days, or lasting four days or more, but not having enough of the symptoms to meet full criteria.

Phase delayed: The condition of having your daily rhythm out of sync with the rising and setting of the sun. Night owls and typically developing adolescents are considered to be phase delayed.

Phototherapy: The use of light to stimulate mood changes.

Presenting symptoms: Signs of discomfort that prompt a visit to a doctor.

Pressured speech: Urgent, non-stop talking that's difficult to interrupt. Pressured speech is a characteristic of hypomania and mania.

Prodromal symptoms: An early sign that may indicate that a psychiatric disorder (including mania or depression) is developing.

Prophylaxis: A fancy word for prevention. Doctors commonly prescribe a maintenance dose of a medication to prevent the onset of symptoms.

Protein kinases: A group of secondary chemical messengers in the neurological system, including the brain, that trigger changes to proteins inside of cells.

Psychiatrist: A physician who specializes in the biology and physiology of the brain. A psychiatrist's role in treating bipolar includes diagnosis and medication prescription as well as patient education and psychotherapy.

Psycho-education: A type of therapy that consists primarily of educating those affected about the condition, its causes, and its treatment so they can more effectively manage the condition.

Psychologist: A professional who specializes in brain development and function, thought processes, emotions, and behaviors. A psychologist can play a vital role in stabilizing moods by assessing brain functions and helping the sufferer adjust negative thoughts and thought processes, regulate emotional responses, and control self-destructive or otherwise maladaptive behaviors.

Psychopharmacology: The study of the effects of medications on the brain.

Psychosis: Brain malfunction that blurs the line between real and imaginary, often causing delusions, auditory hallucinations, and irrational fears.

Psychotropic substance: Any chemical substance (usually a medicine) that affects mental functioning, emotions, or behavior.

Rapid cycling: A state in which mood alternates between depression and mania more than four times in a year.

Repetitive Transcranial Magnetic Stimulation (rTMS): The application of strong, quick-changing magnetic fields to the brain to produce electrical fields indirectly. Researchers are studying it for use in treatment-resistant depression and other disorders.

Schizoaffective disorder: A psychiatric disorder in which symptoms of bipolar disorder and schizophrenia are both present.

Schizophrenia: A psychiatric disorder in which thought becomes dissociated from sensory input and emotions and is accompanied by hallucinations and delusional thinking. Thinking or cognitive skills are also often affected and day-to-day function can be severely impaired. Bipolar is sometimes misdiagnosed as schizophrenia.

Seasonal affective disorder (SAD): A mood disorder that's strongly linked to the change of seasons. People who have SAD commonly experience major depressive episodes in the winter months.

Second messenger systems: Circuits that transmit signals within a brain cell rather than between brain cells.

Selective Serotonin and Norepinephrine Reuptake Inhibitor (SNRI): A class of antidepressant medications that prevent the brain from absorbing and breaking down the neurotransmitters norepinephrine and serotonin after their use. Whether this is the primary mechanism for reducing symptoms of depression is unclear.

Selective Serotonin Reuptake Inhibitor (SSRI): A class of antidepressant medications that prevent the brain from absorbing and breaking down the neurotransmitter serotonin after its use. Whether this is the primary mechanism for reducing symptoms of depression is unclear.

Self-medicate: The attempt to stabilize moods by taking nonprescription chemical substances, including alcohol and marijuana, or by regulating doses of prescription medication without a doctor's assistance.

Serotonin: A neurotransmitter that's a major part of the cellular circuits that regulate mood, anxiety, fear, sleep, body temperature, the rate at which your body releases certain hormones, and many other body and brain processes.

Stigmatize: To brand someone as disgraceful or shameful.

Stressor: Anything that places demands on your brain and body. Stressors are often thought of as negative, but exciting and positive events can also be stressful. Day-to-day life is full of little and big stressors, which the body and brain respond to and then return to baseline. Stress is a necessary and normal part of human function, but certain stressors may contribute to mood instability depending on various other factors.

Support group: A group of patients and/or family members who meet to discuss and empower one another in the face of a common illness.

Tardive dyskinesia: A condition — sometimes caused by the long-term use of neuroleptics — that results in abnormal, uncontrollable muscle movements, often in the mouth and face.

Therapeutic level: The concentration of medicine in the bloodstream required for medication to be effective.

Thyroid: A gland situated below the Adam's apple that produces hormones that control growth, regulate many body functions, and influence moods.

Treatment-resistant depression (TRD): Depression that doesn't respond well to standard medical treatments, including medication.

Tricyclic antidepressant: A class of medications that treat depression and limit the reuptake of the neurotransmitters serotonin and norepinephrine.

Unipolar depression: A mood disorder characterized by episodes of major depression without symptoms of mania or hypomania.

Unspecified bipolar and related disorders: A type of bipolar disorder listed in the fifth edition of Diagnostic and

Statistical Manual of Mental Disorders (DSM-5)that's characterized by hypomanic, manic, or depressive symptoms that cause problems in function, don't fit into any of the other bipolar categories, and can't be attributed to unipolar depression.

Vagus Nerve Stimulation (VNS): Electronic brain stimulation through the vagus nerves in the neck that has some evidence of helping reduces the symptoms of treatment resistant depression (TRD).

Chapter One: Understanding Bipolar Disorder

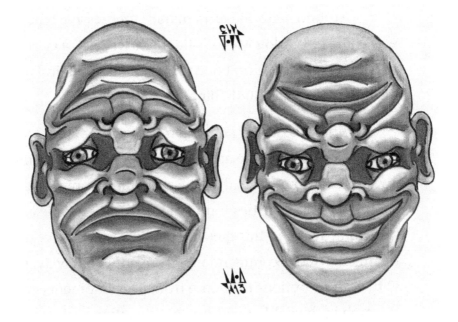

As mentioned earlier, bipolar disorder is formerly known as manic depression, but ancient times particularly during golden years of Ancient Greece, this condition is widely known as melancholia – which is also the original term for depression. Melancholia was derived from "melas" and "chole," which means black and bile respectively.

Other etymologies proposed by early Roman physicians said that the term came from a Greek word "ania" which means producing mental anguish, and "manos" which means excessively loose or relaxing.

Around 1952, the term manic – depressive reaction was coined by Adolf Meyer's book. Karl Kleist, a German psychiatrist, was the first one to call the neurological disorder "unipolar" and "bipolar."

Bipolar disorder since then has evolved, but fortunately through the advances of technology, constant awareness through social media and online communities as well as various charities/foundations, a lot of people are becoming aware of this mental condition, and lots of medical treatments and recommendations are now widely available with various options to choose from. Developments and research in the field of psychology is continuously paving the way to find better treatment solutions for the disorder. Communities online and offline are being formed, and funds are being raised in order to help those who are affected.

Bipolar disorder is both a blessing and a curse; the patient's changing moods can affect their thinking, their relationships and their general outlook in life as well.

However, some famous people who have such condition learned to live with it, and even use it to their advantage.

Facts about Bipolar Disorder

Bipolar disorder causes periods or episodes of abnormal moods or shifting emotional levels. It's a manic – depressive illness that can strike anytime at any given moment. When a person has this kind of brain disorder, they usually experience various symptoms of psychosis which highly depends on the degree or severity of the condition.

Suicidal risks and attempts are the very common among people with a bipolar disorder, especially if they are badly depressed. During those periods, lots of crying, and negativity are involved which is why it is important that people with this disorder are not alone and is always supported by their family and loved ones.

People who are in their 20's are more inclined to attempt suicide, while people between the ages of 30 and 40 years old most often do harm themselves. Anxiety and substance use disorders are usually associated with manic – depression or bipolar disorder.

There are four main types of bipolar disorder; 2 of which are very common (Bipolar I and II disorder), which will be further discuss later on in this book.

Fortunately, you can easily identify if you or any of your loved ones have a bipolar disorder. Common signs are easily being agitated or irritable, always worried or has extreme anxiety, often doing risky things, has suicidal thoughts, or always feeling high or has increased activity levels in an abnormal way.

If for any reason you find yourself constantly changing moods or feeling any abnormal and sudden emotional shifts, you may take some psychological tests or better yet seek professional help. Talking to counselors, and doctors like a psychiatrist can help you manage this condition, or at least help you deal with it.

People with a bipolar disorder will most likely undergo continuous medical treatment especially for severe cases or for those who are always experiencing series of episodes. Therapy is also recommended for patients with this mental condition.

There are also lots of myths about people with bipolar disorder, in the next section, we will bust those myths out for you and give you nothing but facts.

Myths about Bipolar Disorder

To further illuminate what constitutes Bipolar Disorder, it is helpful to know what Bipolar Disorder does not cover. The following are some myths and misconceptions regarding this condition:

Myth #1:

Feeling too high or too depressed is nothing but states of mind. If you for instance are feeling sad, you just need to think positive and shift your focus on something that will make you happy.

Myth Busted:

Bipolar disorder is a real condition that affects the brain, which means that people affected by it can't just simply snap out of their depression or sadness by thinking positively. Although this can help somehow, it's still more complicated than that. It's pretty much like asking a diabetic person to change their blood sugar levels just by changing their state of mind.

Myth #2:

People who undergo psychological treatment are weak because they can't cope up with life's daily struggles.

Myth Busted:

Undergoing treatment should not be regarded as a weakness, in fact it's the complete opposite, people who know in themselves that they are ill and those who seek out medical help are strong and even brave, because they know how to "face their demons, and stare at it in the face." Seeking professional is the best way to learn how to control one's behavior.

Myth #3:

Talk therapy is just pretty much complaining, and it doesn't help.

Myth Busted:

First of all, talking is much better than not communicating at all! Talk therapy has been proven and tested; it is works hand in hand with medications. It is very effective in making the person's behavior stable.

Myth #4:

Medications can change a person's personality, and it can be "addicting" or habit forming.

Myth Busted:

Meds are not addictive if it is properly used and a appropriate dosage is prescribed by a doctor. It does not in any way change a person's personality – personality is innate in every human being. Meds can help modify and manage a mood that's why it shouldn't be compared to drugs or so – called happy pills.

Myth #5:

People with mood disorders will never get better.

Myth Busted:

False! If a person is properly treated, like any other disease or condition, he/she can live a totally normal and stable life. Guess what? Lots of people already do!

Myth #6:

Depression or bipolar symptoms among kids and young adults are normal; it's part of growing old.

Myth Busted:

Such symptoms should be taken seriously especially at a young age. Children can be detected with bipolar disorder even during its infancy, while teenagers or young adults are at high risk for suicidal attempts due to depression. Young people with signs of depression or anxiety should undergo physical examinations.

Myth #7:

People with bipolar disorder or depression can be potentially violent and even dangerous.

Myth Busted:

People with mental illness are not in any way equivalent to being violent or doing acts of violence towards others. In fact, people diagnose with mental illness are even the ones who ends up becoming a victim of violence,

Myth #8:

Bipolar people should consider not having children; it might be passed on to them and could also result to future problems.

Myth Busted:

Like any person who had previous or currently have disorders/diseases may it be mental / emotional or physical can still become a parent. As for the symptoms or possibility of the disorder being inherited by the children, it can most likely be passed on, but it shouldn't be a hindrance for anyone who wanted to have a family. You just need to recognize any signs early on and give them possible treatment as soon as possible. After all, who can better understand them than their parents who are undergoing or have undergone the same thing? Think of it as a bonding experience, and teach your children on how to deal with it the way you did or probably even better.

Myth #9:

Since bipolar people are not mentally stable, they shouldn't be authorize by the government or companies to hold a high position especially in the field of law enforcement

Myth Busted:

If the disorder is properly treated, and the condition is being managed and / or the person is continuously seeking professional help, he/she can and do work at even the highest position possible. The mood disorders don't necessarily affect work performance.

Myth #10:

Only a small percentage of people in the United States commit suicide, it's not a major problem!

Myth Busted:

The fact is suicide is ranking higher than homicide in United States. It is one of the leading causes of death in the country with over 30,000 people a year, 90% of which are believed to be people who have mental disorder. Please do your part to help prevent and lessen this problem.

History of Bipolar Disorder

During the Ancient times in Greece, around the 1st century, physicians back then were already recording symptoms of the bipolar disorder or manic – depression. One of which is Aretaeus of Cappadocia, his notes were unnoticed for many years, but it's one of the earliest records of this diagnosis.

As mentioned earlier, the Greeks and also Romans are the ones who coined the terms "melancholia," which means manic and depressive today. During those times, they also found out that lithium salts can calm people who are hyperactive, and at the same time, also boosting one's energy for those who are depress. Today, believe it or not, lithium is one of the most common treatments for people diagnose with a bipolar disorder.

During the ancient times, people with mental disorders are being executed because they are believed to be possessed by demons. Religious dogmas order mentally unstable people to be put to death. Fortunately through the advancement in medical studies, this kind of practice eventually stopped.

Around 17th century, author Robert Burton, in his book called *The Anatomy of Melancholy,* proposed that music and dancing can be used as a form of treatment for people with melancholia. The medical book also tackled the symptoms as well as possible treatment of what we know today as clinical depression. His book also served as a commentary collection about depression and its effects.

Just a few years after Burton published his book, another author named Theophilus Bonet, wrote a book entitled *Sepuchretum,* and in it he coined the term *manico-*

melancolicus, which is a combination of mania and melancholy. According to him mania and depression are the same kind of mental disorder; his basis was drawn from his autopsy experiences as a doctor, because at that time melancholy and depression are treated as two separate conditions.

Around the 19th and 20th century, Jean-Pierre Falret, a French psychiatrist, published an article around 1851 that was centered on circular insanity. This article was the first ever document about bipolar disorder, that explains details about people shifting from severe sadness to manic excitement. Falret also wrote in his article about the connection of genes among people diagnosed with bipolar disorder. This belief still holds true among medical professionals today.

Around 1921, German psychiatrist known as Emil Kraepelin in his book *Manic Depressive Insanity and Paranoia* broke away from the theory of Sigmund Freud. According to Freud, suppression plays a huge role in society's mental illness. However, Kraepelin did a researched about the biological causes of mental illness, and in his book he discussed in full detail the difference between praecox (now known as schizophrenia) and melancholy. This study continues to be the basis for mental disorder classifications among medical professionals today.

In the early 1950's, another German psychiatrist named Karl Leonhard with his fellow colleagues, discussed the importance of better understanding the classification systems of various mental disorders in order to better treat this kinds of conditions.

During the 1980s, the American Psychiatric Association's (AMA) third revision of *Diagnostic and Statistical Manual of Mental Disorders* (DSM) referred melancholy or manic – depression as "bipolar," that signifies two opposite poles – mania and depression. Thanks to this revision, patients who are diagnosed with manic – depression was not called "maniacs" anymore.

Today now in its 5th revision, the DSM is still the leading manual book that many health professionals and psychiatrist use.

Greek philosopher Aristotle actually acknowledged the condition of melancholy or bipolar disorder because it has become in its own way an inspiration that brought forth to many great artists in history.

Chapter Two: Types of Bipolar Disorder

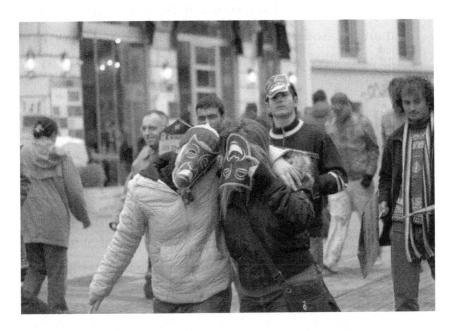

According to AMA's Diagnostic and Statistical Manual of Mental Disorders manuals 5th Revision, there are 4 main types or classifications of bipolar disorder. These are Bipolar I and II, Cyclothymic Disorder, and Rapid – Cycling Bipolar Disorder. In this chapter you will be given an overview of information about the different disorders.

Bipolar I Disorder

Bipolar I disorder is when a person has at least one manic episode or one depressive episode (with or without any previous depressive or manic episode respectively).

Usually patients with bipolar I disorder experienced a depressive episode more than manic episodes. Other clinical or psychotic disorders such as delusional disorder and schizophrenia disorder must not rule out.

It is both common in men and women; usually the first episode that men experience is mania, while in women the first episode is depression.

Bipolar II Disorder

Patients diagnosed with bipolar II disorder usually have more the one depression episodes and also one hypomanic episode. Hypomanic episodes are less severe than manic episodes. A person, who experiences hypomanic sleep less, is very outgoing and has lots of energy; the main difference between hypomanic and manic is that the former is fully functioning and looks completely normal while the latter is experiencing high levels of emotions but may not be properly behaved with others.

People who are hypomanic have no psychosis symptoms and their behavior is not something grandiose or the kind of behavior that will grab everyone's attention. Usually people diagnose with bipolar II disorder is undergoing a major depression. Women are usually affected than men.

Cyclothymic Disorder

Cyclothymic disorder is the milder version of bipolar disorder. People diagnosed with this usually have mood disturbances that have alternate periods of hypomanic episodes, as well as mild to moderate depression.

The baseline for cyclothymia patients is when they feel stable but their moods changes in a snap, and fluctuates. They can experience both mild hypomania, and mild depression. This is like the stage 1 of bipolar disorder, people diagnosed with cyclothymia can experience random but noticeable mood swings within a day or a week.

Rapid-Cycling Bipolar Disorder

Rapid – cycling bipolar disorder also has the same mood swing symptoms, however the difference is that manic and depressive episodes are shorter and rapid, hence its name. The cycles are shorter so the effect it has on people is that manic or depressive states are always changing at a very sudden situation. It is considered the most severe form of bipolar disorder.

This is more common among young people, and affects more women than men. They usually experience more than four episodes of major depression, hypomania, or even mixed symptoms within a day or within a week.

Chapter Three: Phases of Bipolar Disorder

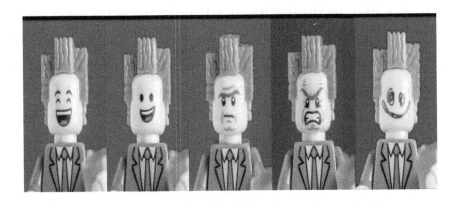

People with bipolar disorder as what you have learned earlier go through lots of emotional ups and downs. The degree of their experiences varies from one person to another. Before learning about the underlying causes of this condition, before learning the signs and symptoms to watch out for, and before you can fully grasp its effect in general, you should first and foremost understand its various phases, so that you'll have an idea on what to do in case you and your loved will experience such episodes.

The most common types are mania and depression, however in some severe cases, mixed episodes, seasonal patterns and rapid cycle also occurs.

Mania

This is probably the upside of having a bipolar disorder, because in a way when the patient is experiencing manic or mania, he/she is in an elevated emotion or he/she is experiencing overwhelming happiness. A person can experience feeling "high" and it includes feelings of confidence, uniqueness, as well as a boosted self – esteem even in hopeless situations.

The downside of mania is that when people experience it, they suddenly feel invincible; their feelings of being "powerful," cloud their judgment, and overestimate their abilities and ideas. The feeling of being "bulletproof or overconfidence" can be used as an advantage if applied to a certain purpose, however this same attitude and overwhelming energy can also somewhat harm them because they are blinded by this feeling and therefore have no concern whatsoever for the actions they will take.

Their ideas and thoughts can become extreme to the point that when they speak about it, no one could actually stop them. Try imagining, sort of like a Eureka moment; it is mostly seen in films where a scientist discovers something like a formula that can change the world. Most of the time, the characters begin talking like a madmen, where no one can interrupt them because their speaking abilities can't even keep up with the thoughts and ideas running through their head. When a person experiences extreme manic episodes, they speak and act like a madmen.

They could exaggerate everything, and could even burst out into singing or dancing spontaneously for no reason at all. It is fun to watch and may be bearable if you are at the privacy of your homes, but if this behavior randomly strikes outside or during events it can be disturbing for others, and can also be dangerous. Hospitalization may be required immediately.

Manic episodes also have psychotic symptoms. Psychosis is simply the state in which a person can't tell what's real and what's not. Simply put, they act like they are high on drugs. Manic people could have hallucinations, false beliefs such as believing that they have superpowers or their identity is different. If you notice that your loved one has these kinds of symptoms, consult a psychologist immediately before it goes out of hand.

Bipolar people experiencing a state of mania can have overflowing energy wherein they only sleep for about 3 hours maximum in a day. Friends and family or anyone in charge of taking care of them could become exhausted because of this overwhelming level of activity.

Depression

Some people would say that everyone at some point of their lives goes through depression. This inevitable state could have many causes or reasons on why it affects people, reasons such as death of a loved one, painful loss, defeat or heartbreaks from a relationship. That feeling could linger on for days, weeks, months and for some people (even those who are completely normal), they could be depress form years.

For patients diagnosed with a bipolar disorder, it is even worse to the point that they can't even get up and they choose to only stay in bed all day. Their mind is moving at a very slow pace, and they don't have interest or would easily lose motivation in any kind of activity. Usually patients undergoing this episode feel like they are worthless creatures, that everything they do are meaningless, that their lives have no purpose. This could actually be potentially dangerous, and it is highly recommended that you always be with the patient during these down moments because it can eventually lead to them taking their own lives. It's important that they have relative or close friends nearby who will never give up on them and will be with them throughout this fleeting episode to avoid any accidents.

Other effects include gaining too much weight over a quick period of time, very low activity level, suicidal thoughts or even suicidal attempts. Like in a manic episode, depressive episodes can also be severe.

Mixed Episode

As what the name suggests, this phase or episode will experience symptoms of mania and depression at the same time. It can often time result to irritability, aggression, hostility and they could also cause harm to other people if not treated properly and immediately. They would usually be prescribed with a medication or may need to stay longer in the hospital to monitor their behavior, and should have a clearance first with a psychologist.

Rapid Cycling

As mentioned earlier, this is the most severe type of bipolar disorder because, the emotions, as the name suggests, quickly and suddenly changes. It is very unpredictable. The only difference between this phase and the mixed episode phase is the period or duration of a certain state of mind or behavior, which is perhaps even more dangerous. This phase also lasts sometimes over a year. The episodes can change from manic to hypomanic then it can change to depressive or a mixed episode over the course of 12 months at a very fast and unpredictable period.

The main reason why it is even more dangerous is because it's much harder to treat. Since their moods are often changing, they can drink a medication for a certain phase but then it could not be quite effective because the state is constantly changing. Usually doctors prescribed various medications for patients that undergo rapid cycling. It is very common among women, especially for those who have thyroid gland problems. Their hormonal imbalance can mimic mania or depression. Around 20% of bipolar patients progresses into rapid cycling.

Seasonal Pattern

Seasonal patterns phase are triggered by a particular season of the year. For instance if a patient only becomes depress at a certain season or period like fall or winter, and their behavior changes back to normal during summer or spring, they most likely have a seasonal pattern depression. The same goes for manic patients with bipolar disorder. They can have a tendency of hypomanic episodes during a particular season.

Depression usually occurs in patients during the months of November, December or January, while suicidal attempts or suicide usually happens around March to May, maybe due to changes in the environment.

Chapter Four: Causes, Diagnosis, and Treatment

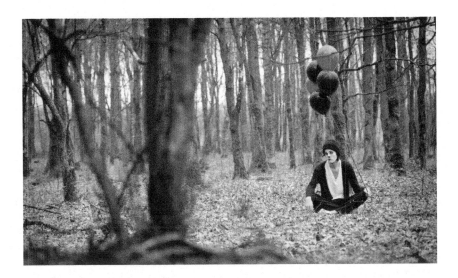

Now that you have an overview of what bipolar disorder is, its types and how it can affect one's mental and behavioral attitudes.

In this chapter you will be given a depth of information about its various causes, common symptoms, diagnosis, prognosis, risk factors, medical treatment as well as other related illnesses. According to scientists, there is no single cause of bipolar disorder. Both biological and environmental factors contribute to this kind of condition and even increase it.

Major Causes of Bipolar Disorder

Most psychotherapists agree that there are three major factors or causes of bipolar disorder, below are risk factors that could have contributed to this illness:

Brain Formation, Structure and Functioning

Research and various scientific studies show the difference between the brain structure of people with bipolar disorder and normal healthy people. There is no reason as to why their brains formed quite different than others, although some may argue that it might be because of indirect factors perhaps during pregnancy, or it may be associated with certain mental disorder that they might have inherited from their parents.

Scientists and doctors in the field of psychology are continuously studying the differences of the brain's functioning of a patient diagnosed with bipolar disorder. It can help them during treatment so that they will be able to know the most appropriate and efficient medication that a particular patient needs.

Genetics

Some medical research suggests that people diagnosed with bipolar disorder have certain genes that tend to develop this kind of mental health condition. However, genes are not the only risk factor that is in play for a person to develop a bipolar disorder. For instance, a study was conducted through examining identical twins; doctors found out that even if one twin developed a bipolar condition, it doesn't mean that the other twin will also have one, despite the main fact that both of them share the exact same genes. However, the genetic makeup of a person can be a large factor that can cause bipolar disorder especially among infants.

Family History

One major cause that could be related as to why certain people have genes that may likely develop a bipolar disorder is due to family history. Usually this kind of condition runs in families. Children with parents or relatives who had bipolar disorder can potentially develop the mental illness compared to children who don't have any family history. However, take note that people who were born in a family with a bipolar disorder history don't usually inherit the condition; it's not absolute that if your parents or relatives are bipolar you will be bipolar too.

Symptoms of a Bipolar Disorder

As you may now know, bipolar disorder can cause a person to have various mood episodes, and usually goes through a rollercoaster of intense emotions, activity levels, behaviors and also has a different sleeping pattern. Whatever type of bipolar disorder you or your family has, you will notice it if you watched out for the following signs:

Signs that a person is going through a Manic Episode:

- Experiencing intensive highs, ups or has an elevated mood
- Has lots of abnormal energy or increased level of activity
- Has feeling of being wired or jumpy or too overwhelmed and excited
- Has a trouble sleeping due to constant change in sleep patterns
- Can become more active than usual
- Can talk really fast about random and unrelated things

- Can be immediately agitated or irritated
- Feels like their thoughts are fast or can't be controlled
- Thinks that they can do lots of different things all at the same time that it could be too overwhelming for a normal person
- Are inclined to do reckless things without thinking about it such as randomly spending lots of money or has abnormal sexual urges.

<u>Signs that a person is going through a Depressive Episode:</u>

- Usually feels sad, very upset, hopeless or has a feeling of emptiness
- Has little to no energy at all
- The level of activity in any interest is fleeting or decreasing
- They either sleep too little or too much
- Can't enjoy the simple pleasures in life
- Is always worried and anxious
- They can't focus or has trouble concentrating over something
- Tend to forget things
- Either eat too little or too much
- Feeling of tiredness even if no strenuous or exhausting activity is being done

- Have suicidal thoughts or have attempted suicide

Symptoms of hypomania are similar to the symptoms of a person with a manic episode, the only difference is that it is milder but it is still noticeable. Even if the person is feeling well or he/she feels like nothing is wrong with, the signs can be obvious and can be recognize by a mentally healthy person. The mood swings and inappropriate level of activity or unusual changes in behavior. If not treated properly or immediately, hypomania will most likely progress to sever manic or depression.

Diagnosis

If you think you or any of your friends and family has been experiencing some signs of bipolar disorder, you may want to consult a psychologist or seek medical help as soon as you can. If bipolar disorder is diagnosed at an early stage or treated properly, you'd be able to deal with it and manage its effects. People who seek professional help live very normal and productive lives.

Before the doctor diagnose you with this mental condition, you may need to complete a physical exam first such as X-rays, CT Scan, blood tests and the like just to rule out other possible conditions. If the mental problem is not caused by any disease or physiological factors such as stress or fatigue, your physician will then conduct a mental health evaluation before referring you to a psychiatrist, sometimes your family doctor or a general doctor can already refer you immediately to a mental health professional so that he/she can conduct the initial mental testing.

Treatment

Treatment is very important for people diagnosed with bipolar disorder because through medical or mental treatment such as therapy, the patient can learn how to manage and gain better control of their mood swings or ever changing emotions as well as other bipolar symptoms.

The most effective treatment procedure includes medication and psychotherapy (also known as talk therapy). Bipolar disorder cannot be completely treated or eradicated; unfortunately it is a lifelong illness. Manic or depressive episodes can come back from time to time even with treatment, some people between episodes are free of mood swings, but for some people have lingering symptoms. The important thing is that even if it is a condition that will last a lifetime, proper and regular treatment can control the bipolar symptoms.

If you are looking to seek medical professional help, then you could choose from a wide range of mental health doctors that specializes in treating bipolar disorders. Some of these doctors are regarded as an expert in a specific form of bipolar condition, it's better to do your research so you can find out more about them and see if you think they can help you. You should opt to go first to your family doctor or a general physician to rule out any other illness and for him/her to also confirm that you might be suffering from a mental illness. Usually your family physician can give you medications to aid in your mood swings; however he or she will also recommend you to go to a psychologist or psychiatrist for further evaluation.

Treatments such as psychotherapy and medications are facilitated and prescribed respectively by a licensed psychologist or in some cases a clinic social worker. During initial diagnosis, you will be ask to do several mental health tests like answering mental health evaluations or through talk therapy so that the doctor can further assess your potential condition as well as its degree.

Most people cope very well with psychotherapy, if you think you or your friends and family are experiencing life – threatening symptoms frequently such as suicidal attempts, substance abuse, aggressive or impulsive behavior, and promiscuity as well as other psychotic symptoms like hallucinations and delusions, then it is highly recommended that you seek a psychiatrist immediately. The degree of the bipolar condition may vary, for some people a psychiatric facility hospitalization may be needed.

Common Medications

Various kinds of medications are a big help to control and manage symptoms of bipolar disorder. That is why it's important to always have a follow – up checkup with your doctor or psychotherapist so that you or your doctor can have a gauge if the current medication is working or not. Appropriate medications are generally used as mood stabilizers, antidepressants, and also include atypical antipsychotics.

Tips before taking any medication:

- Always talk to a legit doctor or pharmacist before taking any medication so that you should be aware of its effects and possible side – effects to the body as well.

- If there are any side – affects you should report it immediately to the doctor so that he or she can change the medicine or maybe give a much appropriate dosage.

- Don't suddenly stop taking any medication without first consulting your doctor, it could lead to a rebound which means that it could worsen the symptoms you are currently feeling. Uncomfortable or serious withdrawal effects are possible if you suddenly stop taking a certain medication without informing your doctor.

Psychotherapy

One of the benefits of going through a therapy aside from taking meds is that it can ultimately guide a patient with bipolar disorder on how to manage his/her condition in a "human level." It can also provide education and support. Patients are given freedom to speak what's on their mind, and their mental or personal issues will be addressed properly with the help of a psychiatrist.

Here are the most common psychotherapy treatments that are used to treat patients with bipolar disorder:

- Cognitive behavioral therapy (CBT)

- Family-focused therapy

- Interpersonal and social rhythm therapy

- Psycho-education

Other Treatments:

- **Electroconvulsive Therapy (ECT)**

This kind of therapy can provide relief especially for people with severe cases of bipolar disorder who were not able to recover from other treatments. ECT is also being used to treat bipolar symptoms for people with other medical condition including women who are pregnant because taking medications can be too risky. However, ECT may also have a short – term side effects such as confusion, memory less, and disorientation. The possible effects or risks of ECT should first be discussed with a health professional.

- **Sleep Medications**

People diagnose with bipolar disorder usually have different sleeping patterns that's why they have trouble sleeping, usually sleeping medications are prescribed to them by their doctors. However, for some people if sleeplessness is not improved even if they have taken sleeping medications, doctors often recommend sedatives.

- **Supplements**

Before taking herbal medications you should first consult it with your doctor. No research studies have been conducted if herbal supplements or natural medicines can help improve the behavior of a bipolar person. Just be careful because since no studies have been conducted yet you won't know if there will be certain side – effects if you take a particular herbal supplement.

- **Life Charts**

As mentioned earlier, even if you are properly or regularly treated, it doesn't mean the the mood swings will completely go away. However, it will likely improve the condition of a patient, if he/she works hand in hand with his/her doctor especially when it comes to managing the symptoms, and discussing any issues that may arise. Keeping a life chart that will document the mood swings, the treatments given, sleep patterns, and important life events can help both the patient and the doctor track their progress, and be able to treat the mental condition effectively.

Prognosis for Bipolar Disorder

Most people diagnosed with bipolar disorder are usually given a combination of medications and scheduled therapy sessions, fortunately most of the time the outcome of these treatments and the responses for medications for many people are positive.

According to a study 50% of people respond well to lithium alone, while around 20 – 30% of people treated with other types of medications also yield an effective result. However, there are still many bipolar people (around 10%) who are not responding well despite being given various medications or other kinds of treatments. Most of them suffer from frequent mood swings and manic – depressive episodes.

On average, bipolar disorder patients are free of symptoms for the first and second episode in about 5 years or so. However, if the treatment is discontinued way too early, it may not be the case. Nevertheless, the results through continuous medication should at least help in improving the interval between mood swings or episodes. According to doctors, a patient will experience an average of 8 – 9 manic or depressive episodes, or mixed mood swings during the course of his or her lifetime.

Bipolar Disorder and Related Illnesses

Some symptoms of bipolar disorder are somewhat similar to other mental illnesses, which of course could make it difficult for the doctor to diagnose. Sometimes, there are people who are experiencing bipolar disorder along with other conditions such as anxiety disorders, substance abuse or even an eating disorder.

Usually people diagnose with bipolar disorders have a higher risk in also experiencing migraine, thyroid gland problems, diabetes, heart diseases, obesity and other physical conditions.

Here are some of the conditions related to bipolar disorder that could also affect the patient's condition.

Pyschosis – this is when a person who has had many episodes of manic – depression are highly at risk. Psychotic symptoms come in the form of hallucinations and delusions. The symptoms tend to match a patient's extreme mood. See example situations below:

- If bipolar patients are experiencing psychotic symptoms during his or her manic episode, then he or she may believe that he/she is very rich, very popular or possess some kind of special powers.

- On the other hand, if bipolar patients are experiencing psychotic symptoms during his or her depressive episode, he/she may believe that he/she committed a hideous crime or may think that his or her life is completely ruined or may think that she is in a kind of extreme poverty situation.

As a result of these combined bipolar and psychotic symptoms, these kinds of people are sometimes misdiagnosed as schizophrenic patients.

Anxiety and ADHD - Anxiety disorders and attention-deficit hyperactivity disorder (ADHD) patients are almost often misdiagnosed among people with bipolar disorder as well.

Substance Abuse – some bipolar patients are mistaken for being a drug abuse because they also tend to use alcohol or dangerous substances which have an impact on their behaviors and attitude. For instance, people think that these patients just can't properly handle relationships or are really terrible with their jobs – then turns to drugs or drinking when things are not going well for them, what friends and family didn't know is that the patient doesn't have a drug or drinking problem, the underlying cause is that it is the effects and symptoms of being bipolar.

Emergency Numbers

If in any way you think you or your loved ones are in crisis, don't hesitate to call the following numbers and reach to the organizations below so that they can help you

- **National Suicide Prevention Lifeline –**
  Call 1-800-273-TALK (8255); available 24 hours a
  day, 7 days a week; calls are all confidential
- **911 Emergency**
- **Nearest hospitals**

Preventive Measures

What to do if you or any of your friends and family is
thinking of harming themselves or having suicidal thoughts:

- Tell what your currently experiencing to other people
  immediately

- Call any licensed medical professional or contact your
  psychiatrist if you already have one

- Go to the nearest hospital immediately or go straight
  to the ER

- If your friend or relative is considering having suicide
  then never leave them alone

- Remove access to guns, knives, or any other potentially harmful tools including medications or substances such as drugs and alcohol

Chapter Five: Other Causes of Bipolar Disorder

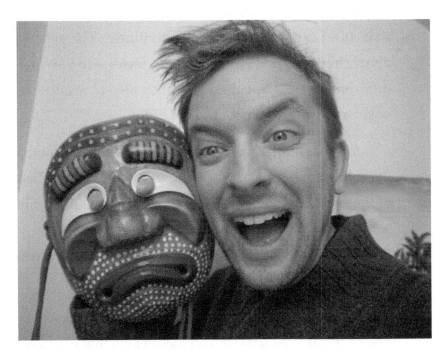

Aside from the common causes mentioned in the previous chapter, there are other underlying causes that are common among patients diagnosed with bipolar disorder. There are neurochemical factors, environmental factors, genetic factors and sometimes it is medication - triggered. In this chapter we will share with you some studies conducted that somehow proves how such factors can result to bipolar disorder.

As what is previously mentioned, there is no one major cause of bipolar disorder, but there are several factors that could cause this mental health illness. The genetic, neurochemical, and environmental factors do vary in different degrees but at the end they also play a role in the onset and progression of the condition.

What many people believe is that the neurobiological disorder that happens in some parts of the brain is because of the malfunction of brain chemicals such as dopamine, serotonin and noradrenaline. But these chemicals lie dormant unless it is activated or triggered by the stresses of life.

Researchers still can't find the exact causes of bipolar disorder but they have found these clues that could play a major role in the advancement of the condition in a person.

Genetic Factors

According to the studies conducted, the families of most people who have bipolar disorder appears to also have some symptoms as well or in one way or another frequently experiences depression. It is believed that this kind of condition is passed from one to another due to genetic lineage. According to researchers, if a parent has a bipolar disorder there is a 15% chance that their child could also develop the same mental condition. If both parents have a history then their offspring could have a 40% chance of inheriting the bipolar disorder. This is the same with identical twins (although it's not always the case), according to the study, if one twin is diagnosed of having a bipolar disorder, there's a 70% chance that the other twin is also bipolar.

The date alone does not prove that the main cause of the condition is just through the genes, other factors should be considered as well like this next one.

Neurochemical Factors

Some studies also show that the bipolar disorder is a biological disorder due to the malfunction of neurotransmitters (also known as chemical messengers) in specific areas of the brain.

Neurotransmitter chemicals includes norepinephrine, and serotonin, however as mentioned earlier, these chemicals may be dormant if it is not in any way triggered by physiological stress or social factors. But it could very well be one of the main causes as well.

Environmental Factors

The environmental factors could also highly be the reason that molds everything together. The trigger of neurochemical factors in a person with genetic disposition could be activated because of different environmental or outside factors.

Even if the person doesn't have the genes of the bipolar disorder condition, its physiological health could suffer and trigger an episode if he/she abuses him/herself with drugs and alcohol or use tranquilizers, which of course started from specific environmental factors such as relationship problems or loss of a loved one.

Environmental and social factors may also result to the apparent changes in the age of occurrence especially if the condition is left untreated in the past. It is usually detected at an early age but could either decrease or progress as time goes on when social factors come into play.

Medication – Triggered Mania

Medications in order to treat bipolar disorder includes antidepressants, however there are times that this very treatment to reduce depression could backfire and can trigger manic episodes for some people. That's why mental health doctors are careful in prescribing antidepressants especially to patients who already had manic episodes, because a depressive mood can become a manic episode if antidepressant drugs are taken.

Anti-manic drugs are then prescribed for these kinds of patients in order to prevent manic episodes; this drug creates sort of a baseline that could partially protect the person from medication – triggered mania caused by antidepressants.

Medications such as appetite suppressants can produce a feeling of highness which resembles that of a manic episode. Such suppressants could trigger high activity levels, abnormal sleep patterns and make the person very talkative or aggressive. Although when the patient stopped taking it, they can return to a normal mood.

Here are some substances than could resemble a manic – like episode:

- Dangerous drugs such as ecstasy, amphetamine, cocaine and other so – called designer drugs.
- Excessive amounts or dosage of over – the – counter drugs such as appetite suppressants and cold preparations or tranquilizers.
- Thyroid meds or non-psychiatric medications such as corticosteroids or prednisone.
- Too much caffeine intake

Various factors such as stress, frequent alcohol or dangerous drugs intake, and sleep deprivation may trigger bipolar episodes especially for people who have a history or have the genes of the condition. Certain medications could also be one of the factors that activates the manic or depressive episodes, that's why it's important to always notify your doctor or psychiatrist about the conditions you've had in the past or your medical history so that your doctor can avoid prescribing you certain medications and prevent unwanted manic episodes.

Chapter Six: Alternative Treatments for Bipolar Disorder

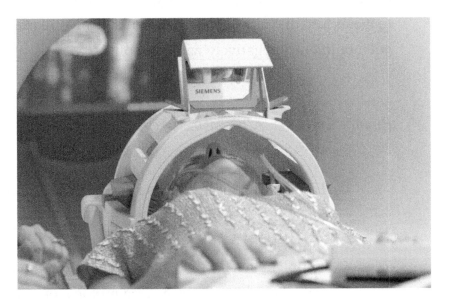

This chapter takes a look at some of the complementary and alternative therapies and treatment that may help persons diagnosed with bipolar disorder. You will also find some unconventional recommendations that may help prevent bipolar disorder, or at least slow its progress.

It should be remembered that no alternative treatments should be considered as a replacement for professional medical advice, and any drugs or pharmaceutical remedies must always be taken after proper consultation, examination, diagnosis and medical prescription by a licensed professional. It is also recommended that any alternative or complementary therapies must only be undertaken with the approval of your medical professional, to make sure that all possible treatments being undertaken will not interact negatively with each other.

Bipolar Disorder Alternative Treatment Tips

- The alternative treatments have extra benefits and can improve the bipolar condition of a patient if it is used with traditional treatments.
- Supplements like fish oil, and herbs like choline can relieve bipolar disorder symptoms or calm the patients down during manic or depressive episodes.
- Maintaining a proper and healthy lifestyle along with alternative therapy treatments can help manage and improve bipolar disorder

According to some patients, alternative treatments like a supplement or herbal medicines relieve them of their bipolar symptoms. Scientific studies have also been conducted to prove how these supplements provide many benefits in order to treat depression or manic episodes. However, further research still needs to be conducted, and some doctors may discourage the use of these alternative medications.

Supplements

There are many studies that show evidences of how herbs and supplements stabilize and improve mood swings and also relieve depression, but it's still important to consult your psychiatrist first before taking in any kind of supplements because it may affect your current treatment or it could cause other side – effects to the body.

Make sure to check first if the supplement is FDA approved or at least produced from a reputable company before buying lots of it. Sometimes the Food and Drugs Administration don't check the quality of such herbal medicines, so better conduct a background check first about its possible effects or the conflict it can potentially cause to your body if it is simultaneously taken with the drugs that your doctor has prescribed.

Below are some of the supplements that so far has been effective in relieving bipolar disorder symptoms.

Fish Oil

Data shows that in countries where fish and fish oil is one of the primary sources of food has less cases of bipolar disorder. Apparently, consumption of seafood is linked to lower cases of bipolar I or bipolar II disorder. This is because fish oil contains Omega – 3 fatty acids.

According to scientific studies, people who are prone to depression have low levels of omega – 3 in their blood. This is why it can also help in improving or treating depression episodes. Omega – 3 fatty acids, also referred to as EPA and DHA, affect the neurochemicals in the brain that are linked to mood disorders.

Consuming at least 1 to 9 grams of fish oil every day may require other supplements before reaching to that level, it may help treat aggression and irritability, it can stabilize the mood conditions, and it can improve brain functions as well as help in reducing depression symptoms.

Children can also take fish oil to increase omega – 3 fatty acids in their bloodstream but it could also cause some side –effects such as heartburn, nausea, bloating, diarrhea, stomach pain or belching. Make sure to consult your physician first.

Rhodiola Rosea

Rhodiola Rosea or also known as golden/arctic root can help in treating mild to moderate depression among bipolar patients. Rhodiola Rosea is a stimulant that can cause insomnia, vivid dreaming or nausea. It's highly recommended to consult with your doctor first especially for people who was previously diagnosed with breast cancer or has a family history of such disease because this arctic root can bind with estrogen receptors which could therefore increase the risk of breast cancer.

S-adenosylmethionine (SAMe)

According to research, SAMe is very effective when it comes to treating depression because it has amino acids that could very well be effective in treating people with bipolar disorder. The main difference between antidepressants and

SAMe is that the former work to boost the brain's production of dopamine, norepinephrine and serotonin, but the latter help balance the neurotransmitters in the brain which in turn also stabilizes a person's mood.

However be careful with SAMe's dosage because it can cause very serious side – effects such as manic episodes, talk to your doctor regarding the proper dosage and also consider its potential effects when it interacts with the current medications you are taking.

Other Herbs and Supplements

Here are some other supplements and herbal medicines that you might want to consider in treating the symptoms of bipolar disorder:

Magnesium

Some studies have shown that taking magnesium supplements can help decrease manic episodes as well as rapid cycling, however further research must be conducted to confirm this findings.

N-acetylcysteine

Taking about 2 grams of N-acetylcysteine once a day can decrease depression and manic episodes and it can also improve the lives of bipolar patients. The reason for this is that this antioxidant alleviates oxidative stress, although according to some studies, it may take about 2 months before seeing its effectiveness.

Choline

Choline is water – soluble vitamin that is reported to be effective when it comes to treating manic symptoms. Most people who take around 2,000 to 7,000 milligrams a day have a certain decrease in manic episodes.

Inositol

This is a synthetic vitamin that could also help in decreasing depressive symptoms, according to studies, about 17% of people diagnosed with resistant depression have significantly improves and recovered after taking this vitamin.

St. John's Wort

So far St. John's Wort has mixed results for people with bipolar disorder, it can somehow only treat short – term to moderate depression. Its extracts are reported to have prevented relapse from an acute depression as well. Make sure to buy a good quality if you choose this kind of alternative medication and discuss with your psychiatrist about its possible side – effects.

Alternative Therapies for Bipolar Disorder

Alternative therapies such as yoga, acupuncture, massage therapy and meditation can help reduce symptoms, and can also reduce anxiety and stress.

For instance, meditation can help a person deal with the various stresses and environmental factors of daily life. Using this kind of therapy can also train you how to control or deal with the world around you. In fact in a survey conducted by researchers, they found out that yoga practitioners diagnose with bipolar disorder live better lives despite their mental condition. Yoga and meditation have positive effects but for some people it can also result to agitation and irritability.

Some people turn to eastern medicine and methods such as acupuncture or Chinese herbal medicines because in many ways it is quite beneficial in relieving anxiety and stress. Acupuncture is a kind of method wherein practitioners insert or poke tiny needles into the body because it improves the flow of energy and the body's balance which also promotes self – healing.

Alternative therapies can't totally cure bipolar disorder, because this condition is incurable, however using these calming techniques can be very helpful in managing one's mood swings, and can also be very valuable in a patient's treatment plan as well.

Other Tech – Based Therapies

Doctors might also recommend patients to undergo through other kinds of therapy (especially for people who may have other physical conditions) aside from the methods mentioned in previous chapters, check them out below:

Light Therapy

Light therapy is mostly used to treat patients with Seasonal Affective Disorder (SAD). This is a kind of depression that is related to a change in seasons. It involves working near a light box that resembles a natural outdoor light; this procedure can improve bipolar disorder. However, it can also trigger manic moods. Consult with your doctor first before undergoing such therapy.

Interpersonal and Social Rhythm Therapy (IPSRT)

The Interpersonal and Social Rhythm Therapy is a kind of psychotherapy that aims to treat people with erratic sleep patterns. Aside from that it can also help the patient to maintain a regular routine, adapt good sleeping habits, and also learn how to solve problems that interrupt their routine.

IPSRT is prescribed along with bipolar disorder medications, because it helps in tracking the patient's mood and managing its lifestyle which in turn could reduce manic and depressive symptoms.

Eye movement desensitization and reprocessing (EMDR)

If a patient with bipolar disorder experiences any traumatic events it can greatly affect and trigger their condition, that's why EMDR was developed. It is a trauma resolution therapy that helps relived emotional and physiological trauma.

The EMDR procedure involves a person thinking about a particular traumatic event or memory in his or her life, as this is being done, the EMDR will then focus on external sensory stimuli such as eye movements and hand taps which can eventually relieve stress and also help a patient process the traumatic experience. Lots of people have so far benefited with EMDR therapy, and it also has significantly improved the bipolar symptoms.

Lifestyle Habits that Can Improve Your Condition

Traditional medications, doctor's recommendations along with alternative treatments can be a huge help in improving a person's bipolar condition, however the lifestyle habits given below can also create more impact during treatment:

- **Regular Exercise** – people with bipolar disorder are at risk of getting diabetes, heart disease and obesity, that's why regular exercise can help prevent such diseases. It also help stabilizes mood swings, cope with depression and improve sleeping patterns.

- **Adequate Sleep** – properly sleeping everyday can reduce irritability and also helps in proper blood circulation. Make sure to get 8 hours of sleep every day.

- **Avoid Unhealthy Relationships** – try avoiding going into complicated and unhealthy relationships or be with people who can be of bad influence to you. Unhealthy behaviors such as frequent alcohol intake and use of illegal substance can trigger worse symptoms of bipolar disorder.

- **Maintain a Proper Diet** – a balanced nutrition will go a long way for your physical and mental conditions. It can help balance out the chemical imbalances in the brain, improve overall health condition, and protect you from further illness. Eating the right foods can ultimately help you improved your bipolar disorder condition.

Important Note:

Most alternative treatments and medications can have side – effects so make sure to consult a physician first before doing anything. Aside from that, your insurance may also not cover these treatments and therapies, so better be prepared financially, such procedures may be expensive.

Chapter Seven: The Future of Bipolar Disorder

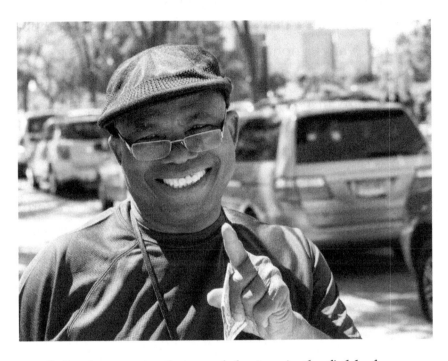

Scientists, researchers and doctors in the field of mental health had evolved in terms of knowledge and treatments in order to manage patients with bipolar disorder. The advent of technology, and the educational advancement helped modern science propelled to staggering heights especially in terms of discoveries and various kinds of treatments; we've come a long way in just the past century if you think about it. However, the continuous development and research is still something every student of medicine – whether they are a medical practitioners, general physicians or mental health specialists, as well as scientists – needs to do so that people diagnose with this condition can have various options (especially when it comes to treatments), more accurate knowledge than ever, and possibly inspire hope and the possibility of a long – term cure to those who were diagnosed with severe cases.

Bipolar disorder usually appears to people on their 20's, however it can already be detected at a very early age, and it can also be triggered at any stage of life. The most important thing is to recognized the tell – tale signs as early as you can so that you or your loved can be given treatment as soon as possible. The earlier the diagnosis, the earlier the treatments will be given, which in turn would be beneficial to the patients and to their families in the long run.

In this chapter, we will share with you the present challenges and struggles of mental health doctors on how to effectively treat the condition as well as what the future may hold for patients with bipolar disorder – the possible technology – based treatments, new medical approaches, and how science can harness today's advanced technology in order to find a cure to the condition. We also provided you with Frequently Asked Questions at the last pages of the book.

Current Challenges

Before we tackle on the future of bipolar disorder and its possible advance treatments, we should take a look first at the challenges that this condition currently face. Doctors and medical researchers look at the current situation on how they treat their patients today because this will serve as a guide on how to improve such treatments or therapies in the future.

The most challenging problem that doctors faced today is accurate diagnosis and proper treatments. Mental health professionals and even specialists sometimes can't pinpoint the actual condition because the symptoms for bipolar disorder are very similar to other mental health conditions such as schizophrenia, anxiety disorders, or ADHD. If a doctor inaccurately diagnoses the condition or the type of bipolar disorder, there's a huge risk on the treatment that will be given to the patients. Until today, even with proper medical knowledge, it's still a hit and misses for the doctors.

According to Dr. Goodwin from George Washing University Medical Center, bipolar disorder is often times misdiagnosed as unipolar depression simply because the symptom that is first seen by the doctors is depression instead of mania. He also noted that when bipolar disorder patients consulted with a psychiatrist for the first time, and if they were asked regarding the pattern or frequency of their depressive or manic episodes most of them can't also accurately identify those periods – which of course makes it harder to diagnose. Unlike if a person, say for example has a heart disease or is stricken with cancer, the symptoms are very easy to identify because it shows physically compared to mental disorders.

Dr. David Kemp together with his colleagues conducted a study in which they gathered patients both from private hospitals and community clinics who was diagnosed with depression. What they did was assessed these patients to see if they have bipolar symptoms using a questionnaire called the Mood Disorders Questionnaire (MDQ); it has 73% sensitivity and can identify signs of bipolar disorder.

Almost 92% of the patients recruited are identified with bipolar disorder. The analysis also revealed that the factor which could predict MDQ score is the patient's perception that people were unfriendly. Factors that can predict positive MDQ scores also include comorbid anxiety disorder, previous depression diagnosis in the last 5 years, family history of bipolar disorder, and a history of legal problems

There's a 40% chance of being positive for mood disorder if the patient scores three out of the five predictive factors mentioned. The study also found out that having a history of multiple antidepressant failure is not a factor.

Impacts of Misdiagnosed Condition

As what is previously mentioned, if bipolar disorder is left untreated, it can result to severe cases and yields a higher rate of suicide. According to the National Institute of Mental Health, about 2.4 million Americans every year are diagnosed with bipolar disorder, that's why misdiagnosis is actually a significant problem. The suicide rates among these patients are 20 times than the rest of the population.

It can be potentially lifesaving if the disorder is accurately diagnosed and if it's just on time. According to Dr. Goodwin, the selection of appropriate treatment and management presents another major challenge given the misdiagnosis for bipolar patients.

Antidepressants can destabilize bipolar illnesses because it is fairly well – established but the long term benefits of these meds have yet to be proven.

Depression, according to Dr. Goodwin, can be much more difficult to manage especially when treating bipolar diseases. In fact almost two – thirds of bipolar disorder patients usually undergo depressive states. Lithium still remains to be the most essential therapeutic medication in managing the symptoms of bipolar disorder. Another medication that is very helpful in treating the disorder is called Lamictal, it has been proven that it even has better antidepressant effect, and Dr. Goodwin even suggested the possibility of combining the efforts of both drugs to combat depressive and manic symptoms.

Doctors in the field of psychology is continuously finding ways on how to accurately diagnose a possible bipolar disorder condition, and with the help of technology they are pretty confident in time they'll be able to use such advancements for proper diagnosis.

Long – Term Maintenance

Another major challenge is keeping patients on the long term therapy required to treat the condition and properly manage it.

According to Dr. Holly Swartz, various pharmacologic and treatment strategies promise greater efficacy in bipolar disorder, only when treatment adherence is high, and according to her that is a huge challenge. Lots of factors are involved that affects the treatment adherence such as the patient's age, gender, educational attainment, marital status as well as psychiatric comorbidities.

Dr. Swartz also added that the side effects of some medications are very common, which could also be the reason why bipolar patients do not take 30% of the doses prescribed to them. The satisfaction of the patients always affects adherence, it is highly correlated with the treatment outcomes.

Some studies also found out those patients who are satisfied with providers usually have better attitudes towards their conditions than patients who are unsatisfied, which is why therapeutic alliance is also an important predictor of patient satisfaction because it can lead to better treatment outcomes.

Researchers also found out that the main factors that could predict in making the patients stay well or better deal with the disorder is if they accepted diagnosis, education, awareness, recognizing trigger factors, and discovering warning signs early on.

Some of the tips that a patient could do according to many mental health doctors include sleeping well, being able to handle stress properly, acquiring treatment, being involved in a support group or having lots of support from friends and family, and maintaining discipline when it comes to following the doctor's treatment plan or recommendations.

According to Dr. Swartz, if a doctor can help his/her patient in monitoring their moods, and properly educate them, they can be satisfied with the results and could be more inclined to maintain their treatment or therapies.

Newly Approved Medications

Zyprexa (olanzapine) and Abilify (aripiprazole) are two of the newly FDA approved meds to treat bipolar disorder. Dr. Goodwin further explained that these meds were based on the results of 12 month trials, that one year trial only indicates that those drugs prevent a backfire or a relapse back into an episode a patient has recovered from. Its maintenance effect are proven and tested.

Another drug that is currently being tested is called Seroquel (quetiapine). This drug can potentially become both an antidepressant and antimanic medicine for acute settings. Even if this med is still undergoing further evaluation, it could be a very effective treatment for acute depressive states, and can also be used as long – term prophylaxis against depression.

Future Bipolar Disorder Diagnosis and Treatments

Now that you've learned the challenges that bipolar disorder is currently facing, it's now time to focus on its possibilities especially now that there are lots of technological advancements that can be beneficial to the patients and the doctors as well.

In this section, we will discuss some of the equipment that can now be used in order to detect early signs of bipolar disorder and also give you a glimpse of the possible future treatments including new forms of psychotherapies.

The Future of Bipolar Disorder Diagnosis

A recent study has shown that using an Magnetic Resonance Imaging or commonly known as MRI can be very effective when it comes to detecting a mental illness including bipolar disorder or other psychotic symptoms.

Researchers were still trying to find out a way on how to maximize MRI's benefits in order to properly distinguish bipolar patients from a mentally normal person through the use of brain scans and other analysis data.

As what is mentioned earlier, one of the major challenges of this disorder especially for doctors is early detection and proper diagnosis, in some cases, it almost takes over 10 years before making an accurate diagnosis, making bipolar disorder among the top 10 disability cases in the world.

Dr. Frangou and her team of medical mental practitioners, tried several tests in using MRI to scan patients who are healthy, and those who have bipolar disorder, using various computational models, the experiment was a success. It correctly identified people with bipolar disorder and normally healthy people with 73% accuracy using brain scans alone!

They replicated this experiment and the results were almost the same, which means that MRI can help in diagnosing a patient in a short period of time. If this is further evaluated and proven, along with other possible high – tech equipment, diagnosis could be easy and treatment can be given immediately to bipolar patients, which in turn can save lots of lives.

Diagnosis is currently identified only through self – reporting from patients and observation using a set of scientifically – defined symptoms, this kind of approach is also vital in terms of building relationships between the doctor and their patients, it can also be a means of support that patients need, and can also encourage practice of awareness on the part of the bipolar person. This kind of approach alongside using machineries like the MRI can significantly detect the condition very early on.

According to Dr. Frangou, although their research is still under evaluation, it can create a major shift in the way psychologists approached diagnosis in psychiatry.

The Future of Bipolar Disorder Therapies

Scientists remained on the lookout for new forms of therapies that can aid the mood swings of bipolar patients. Current medications can reduce symptoms but it's not long – term, they don't get well, that's why therapy is also recommended along with medications.

One of the new forms of therapies that significantly improved bipolar patients who were depress is a brain scan called Echo-Planar Magnetic Resonance Spectroscopic Imaging (EP-MRSI). According to researchers, the EP – MRSI have shown much improvement in a patient's mood swing (30%) compared to using MRI. Researchers are now speculating that the benefit could be coming from the electric fields that are being induced by the scan. Now, doctors are attempting to incorporate scanning as part of treating the patients. Another type of scan that could also have a potential is called Transcranial Magnetic Stimulation; studies are still on – going for this possible therapeutic forms.

Stem Cell to Treat Bipolar Disorder

A study is now being conducted by researchers in the University of Michigan about using stem cell in order to treat people suffering from bipolar disorders.

Researchers took a cell from bipolar patients, and turned those cells into neurons, and then they compared those neurons to the cells of healthy people who are not bipolar. What they found out is that bipolar cells communicate and behaved differently than those of normal healthy cells. These neurons responded differently to lithium as well. Turning a cell into neurons using the skin of the bipolar patients made it possible to look at how these neurons from those who were diagnosed with the disorder responded to medications.

This addresses one of the major problems that doctors faced today regarding the illness since they can't predict the reaction or response of patients to medical treatment or there is no existing method to determine if the medication given will be effective or not. Using stem cells from a patient can paved a major shift when it comes to providing the proper medication during mood swings without risking the patients' well – being. If the stem cell research is a success, doctors can just grab a sample from a particular patient, then study that specific cell, and try testing it with different medications to know the reactions or response; thus, finding a much more accurate, appropriate and effective treatment but not at the expense of the patient.

Stem cells are very unique because it has the genetic code for various types of cells in the body, that's why scientists can use it to grow neurons or even develop an entire organ. They can also reprogram the skin cell into a stem cell. For bipolar patients what this can do is to basically allow the doctors to see their patient's brain inside out in order to recommend a better treatment or prescribed an appropriate medication.

Once these new methods of treatments and new medication discoveries are proven and approved, the future certainly looks bright for patients diagnosed with bipolar disorder. There may not be a cure at the moment, but through continuous research, experiments, and technological innovations of dedicated scientists and doctors, there could be a hope for finding one!

Bonus Chapter:

From History to Hollywood:

Famous People Who Have Bipolar Disorder

Bipolar disorder is a mental condition that can affect one's life negatively. It's an incurable disorder that one has to endure in his/her lifetime. However, for some people they learned how to manage and deal with their untreatable condition, and use it to their advantage.

In this bonus chapter, you will get to know some of the most famous Hollywood celebrities and people in history who were diagnosed with a bipolar disorder, but still somehow were able to make it big and achieved incredible feats despite their condition. And although, for some of them the disorder took a toll in their lives, for the most part it didn't stop them from becoming who they wanted to be; in fact it brought out the best in them, this just goes to show that despite of the struggles, anyone can live a an amazing life as long as you will it.

Notable Hollywood Celebrities with Bipolar Disorder

1. Carrie Fisher

History: Before her recent death, Fisher admitted that she is diagnosed with bipolar disorder; she was on 7 medications but that didn't stop her from conquering her dark side.
Profession: Spokesperson, Novelist, Screenwriter, Actor, Script doctor, + more
Known For: Star Wars: Episode IV - A New Hope, Star Wars: Episode V - The Empire Strikes Back, Star Wars: Episode VI - Return of the Jedi, Star Wars: Episode VII - The Force Awakens

2. Marilyn Monroe

History: Monroe died in 1962 due to probable suicide; it was reported that she was facing drastic mood changes and was undergoing emotional problems. Nevertheless, she still made her mark in Hollywood.
Profession: Film Producer, Model, Actor, Singer, Showgirl
Known For: Some Like It Hot, The Seven Year Itch, Gentlemen Prefer Blondes, How to Marry a Millionaire

3. Amy Winehouse

History: She was diagnosed with bipolar disorder and she used self – medications such as drugs and alcohol. She died in 2011 due to alcohol poisoning. She was one of the best musicians in the world.

Profession: Arranger, Musician, Singer-songwriter

Known For: About Time, The Great Gatsby, Amy, Life as We Know It

4. Kurt Cobain

History: It was unknown if Nirvana singer Kurt Cobain was officially diagnose with the disorder, but according to his close friends he suffered from this condition. He committed suicide in 1994. Nevertheless, he is one of the reasons why Nirvana became one of the most famous bands in the world.

Profession: Guitarist, Songwriter, Musician, Singer, Artist

Known For: Moulin Rouge! Jerry Maguire, The Big Short, Jarhead

5. Frank Sinatra

History: According to sources, Sinatra constantly experienced lots of mood swings both a manic and depressive episodes, despite his condition he managed to become one of the most renowned singers in the 50s throughout the 60's. He died at the age of 83.

Profession: Conductor, Film Producer, Actor, Singer

Known For: From Here to Eternity, Ocean's 11, The Manchurian Candidate, The Man with the Golden Arm

6. Demi Lovato

History: When Demi Lovato found out about her diagnosis, she was quite relieved because according to her, she's not crazy after all and that there's a medical reason for it. She started in Disney Channel with the Jonas Brothers before becoming a recording artist; she is now a judge in the X-Factor, and has appeared in many shows.

Profession: Musician, Singer-songwriter, Actor, TV Personality, Dancer

Known For: The X Factor, Frozen, Princess Protection Program, Camp Rock

7. Axl Rose

History: Although Rose contradicted his bipolar diagnosis, the symptoms of the disorder are highly noticeable. He is the lead vocalist of Guns N Roses – one of the greatest rock bands in the 80's.

Profession: Record producer, Guitarist, Musician, Singer-songwriter, Film Producer, + more

Known For: (Vocalist) Guns N Roses, Terminator 2: Judgment Day, The Wrestler, Terminator Salvation, Gone Baby Gone

8. Mike Tyson

History: The former world champion had been diagnosed with bipolar disorder and he is also quite recently been struggling with drugs and alcohol. He has since received treatment and is now sober. His condition didn't stop him from becoming a famous boxer and the Undisputed World Heavyweight Champion.

Profession: Film Producer, Actor, Athlete, Professional Boxer

Known For: Tyson, The Hangover, The Hangover Part II, Rocky Balboa

9. Ted Turner

History: CNN founder, Ted Turner, was diagnosed with bipolar disorder in the 80s, and he was given lithium for his treatment. He is one of the most influential personalities in the media industry.

Profession: Businessperson, Television producer, Entrepreneur, Film Producer, Screenwriter, + more

Known For: Cable News Network, Turner Broadcasting System, Captain Planet and the Planeteers, WCW Monday Nitro, Captain Planet and the Planeteers, Portrait of the World USSR

10. Jean Claude Van Damme

History: Martial artist, Van Damme, is claiming that his cocaine addiction was because of his bipolar disorder. Nevertheless, his work and contribution as one of Hollywood's martial artist and action superstar made him famous.

Profession: Film Producer, Screenwriter, Film Editor, Actor, Martial artist, + more

Known For: Double Impact, Universal Soldier, Kickboxer, Bloodsport

Notable People in History with Bipolar Disorder

1. Edgar Allan Poe

History: According to sources, Poe always evoked in his writings of him experiencing or interacting with his "double self." He's one of the greatest writers and poet in American Literature

Profession: Magazine editor, Poet, Literary critic, Novelist, Author, + more

Known For: Tales of Terror, Witchfinder General, The Pit and the Pendulum, The Masque of the Red Death, The Raven

2. Abraham Lincoln

History: He was not formally diagnosed with the disorder but many historians believe that the president suffered from this condition. He became the 16th President of the United States, and is regarded as one of the greatest presidents and politicians in American History.

Profession: Statesman, Politician, Lawyer

Known For: President of the United States, The Perfect Tribute, Atlanta Symphony Golden Anniversary, A Tribute to John F. Kennedy from the Arts, Lincoln's Gettysburg Address

3. Ernest Hemingway

History: One of the famous novelists of the 20th century had manic – depressive episodes and he was treated using electroshock therapy back then.

Profession: Journalist, Novelist, Author
Known For: To Have and Have Not, The Killers, A Farewell to Arms, For Whom the Bell Tolls

4. Vincent Van Gogh

History: According to many historians, the painter's changing moods and extreme personality are signs that he struggled with bipolar disorder. He was one of the acclaimed painters in history.
Profession: Painter, Artist
Known For: The Starry Night painting, Café Terrace at Night, The Potato Houses, Irises

5. Ludwig van Beethoven

History: According to many historians and biographers, Beethoven suffered from this mental condition. What's interesting is how he turned that to his advantage to become one of the acclaimed composers of all time.

Profession: Songwriter, Pianist, Musician, Lyricist, Composer, + more

Known For: Django Unchained, A Clockwork Orange, The King's Speech, The Pianist

6. Charles Dickens

History: One of the greatest authors in history was also believed to have suffered from bipolar disorder. Nevertheless the condition didn't hinder him in creating great novels and classic literature in Europe.

Profession: Novelist, Author, Writer, Playwright

Known For: A Christmas Carol, Scrooged, Oliver!, Great Expectations

7. Sir Isaac Newton

History: According to many historians, Newton is very aggressive yet insecure; he was believed to have a bipolar condition because of his rages. His passion and "fire" lead

him to discovering many scientific breakthroughs that made him one of the most influential scientists of all time.
Profession: Mathematician, Physicist, Chemist, Scientist, Philosopher
Known For: Newtonian mechanics, Universal gravitation, Calculus, Newton's laws of motion, Optics

8. Florence Nightingale

History: She was also known for having bipolar disorder symptoms according to many historians.
Profession: Nurse, Statistical graphics, Nursing, Writer, Statistician
Known For: Pioneering Modern Nursing

9. Jackson Pollock

History: According to many biographers, Pollock exhibited all symptoms of bipolar disorder condition. He is a famous American painter and a major figure in abstract expressionism.
Profession: Painter
Known For: Autumn Rhythm Number, Blue Poles, Number 1 (Lavander Mist)

10. Jack London

History: His erratic moods and heavy drinking is due to untreated bipolar conditions according to historians. He is an American novelist and social activist, and one of the pioneers of science fiction.

Profession: Journalist, Sailor, Novelist, Screenwriter, Author

Known For: White Fang, The Call of the Wild, Queen of the Yukon, Two Men of the Desert, The Assassination Bureau

Index

H

I

L

M

N

O

P

R

S

T

V

Photo References

Page 1 Photo by Laura Taylor via Flickr.com,
<https://www.flickr.com/photos/bookgrl/2335948626/>

Page 25 Photo by MrModiant via Flickr.com,
<https://www.flickr.com/photos/mrmodiant/11437070965/>

Page 40 Photo by Vladimer Shioshvili via Flickr.com,
<https://www.flickr.com/photos/vshioshvili/403391656/>

Page 45 Photo by clement127 via Flickr.com,
<https://www.flickr.com/photos/clement127/12038911053/>

Page 53 Photo by Jorn Idzerda via Flickr.com,
<https://www.flickr.com/photos/jornidzerda/6938919650/>

Page 72 Photo by Berewin via Flickr.com,
<https://www.flickr.com/photos/berewin/8365696548/>

Page 79 Photo by Penn State via Flickr.com,
<https://www.flickr.com/photos/pennstatelive/9502139857/>

Page 93 Photo by Caleb Woods via Flickr.com,
<https://www.flickr.com/photos/calebwoods10/11767919503/in/photolist>

References

9 Natural Therapies for Bipolar Depression –
everydayhealth.com
<http://www.everydayhealth.com/bipolar-
disorder/alternative-treatments-for-bipolar-disorder.aspx>

**APA: Diagnostic and Treatment Challenges in Bipolar
Disorder Remain** – MedPageToday.com

http://www.medpagetoday.com/psychiatry/bipolardisorder/
3735

Bipolar Disorder's Basic Fact Sheet – Healthline.com
http://www.healthline.com/health/bipolar-disorder/fact-
sheet?ref=tc

Bipolar Disorder: Causes, Symptoms, and Treatments –
Medical News Today

http://www.medicalnewstoday.com/articles/37010.php

Bipolar Disorder Overview – Webmd.com
http://www.webmd.com/bipolar-disorder/

Bipolar Disorder – National Institute of Mental Health
https://www.nimh.nih.gov/health/topics/bipolar-disorder/index.shtml

Bipolar Disorder – Mayoclinic.org
http://www.mayoclinic.org/diseases-conditions/bipolar-disorder/home/ovc-20307967

Bipolar Disorder – Healthline.com
http://www.healthline.com/health/bipolar-disorder

Bipolar I disorder – Wikipedia.org
https://en.wikipedia.org/wiki/Bipolar_I_disorder

Causes of Bipolar Disorder – PsychCentral.com
https://psychcentral.com/disorders/bipolar/bipolar-disorder-causes/

Myths and Facts about Depression and Bipolar Disorder – DBSAlliance.org

http://www.dbsalliance.org/pdfs/mythsfinal.pdf

Diagnosis of the Future? Brain Scan Shows Promise in Diagnosing Bipolar – PsychCentral.com

https://psychcentral.com/news/2013/06/09/diagnosis-of-the-future-brain-scan-shows-promise-in-diagnosing-bipolar/55793.html

Emerging Bipolar Therapies – Psychcentral.com

https://psychcentral.com/lib/emerging-bipolar-therapies/

First Stem Cell Study of Bipolar Disorder Hints At A Future Of Better, More Effective Treatments – Bustle.com

https://www.bustle.com/articles/19203-first-stem-cell-study-of-bipolar-disorder-hints-at-a-future-of-better-more-effective-treatments

Frequently Asked Questions: Bipolar Disorder - MoodDisorders.ca

https://www.mooddisorders.ca/faq/bipolar-disorder

Genetics and Neurobiology: The Future of Bipolar Disorder Treatment and Diagnosis – MedicalDaily.com

http://www.medicaldaily.com/genetics-and-neurobiology-future-bipolar-disorder-treatment-and-diagnosis-245749

Glossary of Bipolar-Related Terms – Dummies.com
http://www.dummies.com/health/mental-health/glossary-of-bipolar-related-terms/

List of Famous People with Bipolar Disorder – Ranker.com
http://www.ranker.com/list/famous-people-with-bipolar-disorder/celebrity-lists

New Approach Leads toward More Effective Bipolar Treatments – BBRFoundation.org
https://bbrfoundation.org/discoveries/new-approach-leads-toward-more-effective-bipolar-treatments

Phases of Bipolar Disorder – PsychCentral.com
https://psychcentral.com/lib/phases-of-bipolar-disorder/

Rapid Cycling in Bipolar Disorder – webmd.com
http://www.webmd.com/bipolar-disorder/guide/rapid-cycling-bipolar-disorder#1-4

The 5 Biggest Challenges of Bipolar Disorder – everydayhealth.com

http://www.everydayhealth.com/hs/bipolar-
   depression/challenges-of-bipolar-disorder/

The Courses of Bipolar Disorder Over Time –
   everydayhealth.com
http://www.everydayhealth.com/bipolar-disorder/bipolar-
   disorder-prognosis.aspx

The Challenges of Accurately Diagnosing Bipolar Disorder
   – Health.com
http://www.health.com/health/condition-
   article/0,,20275016,00.html

The History of Bipolar Disorder – Healthline.com
http://www.healthline.com/health/bipolar-disorder/history-
   bipolar?ref=tc

What is Bipolar Disorder? – Healthline.com
http://www.healthline.com/health/bipolar-disorder/famous-
   creative-people?ref=tc

Who Gets Bipolar Disorder? – psychcentral.com
https://psychcentral.com/lib/who-gets-bipolar-disorder/

.

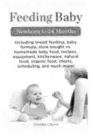

Feeding Baby
Cynthia Cherry
978-1941070000

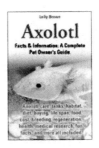

Axolotl
Lolly Brown
978-0989658430

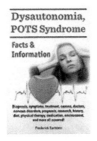

Dysautonomia, POTS
Syndrome
Frederick Earlstein
978-0989658485

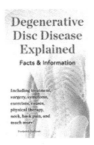

Degenerative Disc
Disease Explained
Frederick Earlstein
978-0989658485

Sinusitis, Hay Fever,
Allergic Rhinitis Explained
Frederick Earlstein
978-1941070024

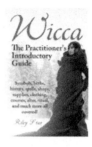

Wicca
Riley Star
978-1941070130

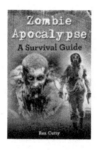

Zombie Apocalypse
Rex Cutty
978-1941070154

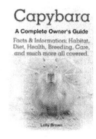

Capybara
Lolly Brown
978-1941070062

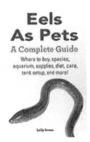

Eels As Pets
Lolly Brown
978-1941070167

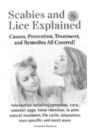

Scabies and Lice Explained
Frederick Earlstein
978-1941070017

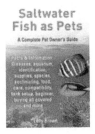

Saltwater Fish As Pets
Lolly Brown
978-0989658461

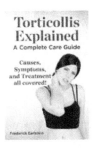

Torticollis Explained
Frederick Earlstein
978-1941070055

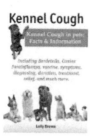

Kennel Cough
Lolly Brown
978-0989658409

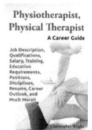

Physiotherapist, Physical
Therapist
Christopher Wright
978-0989658492

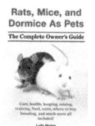

Rats, Mice, and Dormice
As Pets
Lolly Brown
978-1941070079

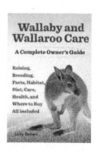

Wallaby and Wallaroo Care
Lolly Brown
978-1941070031

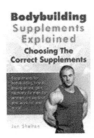

Bodybuilding Supplements
Explained
Jon Shelton
978-1941070239

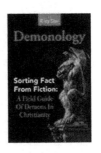

Demonology
Riley Star
978-19401070314

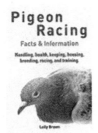

Pigeon Racing
Lolly Brown
978-1941070307

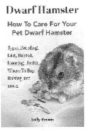

Dwarf Hamster
Lolly Brown
978-1941070390

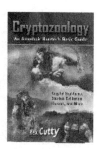

Cryptozoology
Rex Cutty
978-1941070406

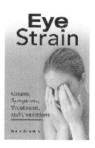

Eye Strain
Frederick Earlstein
978-1941070369

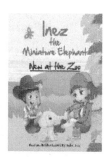

Inez The Miniature Elephant
Asher Ray
978-1941070353

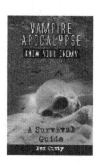

Vampire Apocalypse
Rex Cutty
978-1941070321

Bipolar Disorder Explained   P a g e | **138**

Made in the USA
Middletown, DE
17 November 2020

24326343R00086